Nourishing Recipes for Cancer Patients

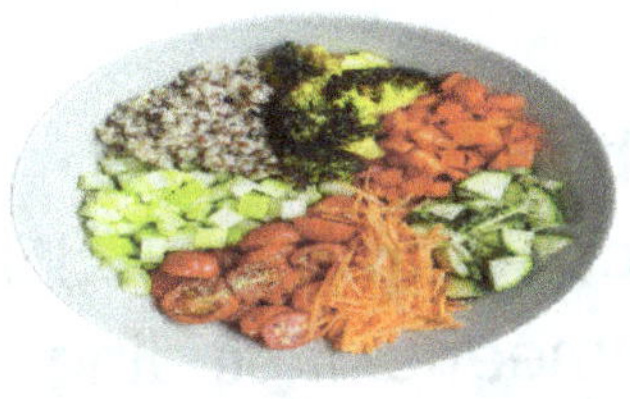

A Guide to Cancer-Friendly Food and Wine

Priscilla J. Schulz

Introduction

Welcome to "Food and Wine for Cancer Patients: Nourishing Recipes and Preparation Tips." This comprehensive guide aims to provide cancer patients, caregivers, and anyone interested in cancer-friendly nutrition with a wealth of valuable information and resources. We understand the importance of a well-balanced and nourishing diet during cancer treatment and recovery, and this book is designed to empower you with the knowledge and inspiration to make informed food choices that support your overall health and well-being.

Chapter 1 delves into the critical role of nutrition in cancer care. We explore how dietary choices can impact treatment outcomes and delve into the specific nutritional needs during cancer treatment. Additionally, we address common eating challenges faced by patients and provide practical strategies to overcome them.

Chapter 2 focuses on building a cancer-friendly pantry. We guide you through stocking nutrient-rich staples and selecting optimal food choices that align with your health goals. Learn about healthful cooking oils and ingredients that can enhance the nutritional value of your meals.

In Chapter 3, we present a range of wholesome breakfast options that provide nourishment and energy to start your day on the right note. From nutrient-packed smoothies and shakes to energizing breakfast bowls and whole-grain ideas, these recipes are designed to support your well-being.

Chapter 4 explores the comforting world of nourishing soups and healing broths.

Discover immune-boosting vegetable soups, comforting bone broths, and creamy pureed soups that cater to sensitive palates, providing sustenance and comfort during your cancer journey.

Flavorful main courses take the spotlight in Chapter 5, offering protein-rich poultry and seafood dishes, along with delectable plant-based alternatives and whole grain meals that provide strength and vitality.

Chapter 6 introduces you to nutrient-dense salads and side dishes. Fresh and colorful salad combinations, wholesome grain and legume salads, and vegetable side dishes with a twist will bring joy to your table while nourishing your body.

In Chapter 7, we focus on managing eating challenges during cancer treatment. Coping with taste changes, loss of appetite, and dealing with nausea and digestive discomfort are essential aspects we address to help you find joy in your meals.

For those with a sweet tooth, Chapter 8 offers a delightful selection of indulgent and nourishing desserts. From healthful sweet treats to fruit-forward desserts with a touch of decadence, we prove that desserts can still be enjoyed during your journey.

In Chapter 9, we explore food and wine pairings for cancer patients, enhancing mealtime with sensory experiences and mindful consumption. Learn to create a calming environment for mealtime and incorporate gentle exercise and movement to promote well-being.

Finally, Chapter 10 discusses nurturing the mind-body connection. We emphasize the importance of mindfulness in food preparation and consumption, highlighting how it complements your cancer journey. Discover how to create a calming environment during mealtime and incorporate gentle exercises that support your overall health.

Throughout this book, we encourage you to embrace the power of food as a tool to nurture your body, mind, and spirit. Every recipe, tip, and resource is carefully curated to help you make thoughtful choices that promote your well-being during this transformative time. Remember, you are not alone on this journey, and we are here to support you every step of the way. Let's embark on this culinary adventure together, embracing nourishing recipes and preparation tips that elevate your quality of life and enhance your journey through food and wine.

CHAPTER ONE

Understanding the Role of Nutrition in Cancer Care

1. The Impact of Diet on Cancer Treatment Outcomes

The influence of nutrition on cancer treatment results may be considerable. A nutritious and balanced diet may assist support the body throughout cancer treatment, promote general well-being, and aid in controlling treatment side effects. Certain foods, such fruits, vegetables, and whole grains, supply critical minerals and antioxidants that enhance the body's capacity to fight cancer and recover from therapy.

It's vital for cancer patients to collaborate with healthcare specialists, such as oncologists and registered dietitians, to build tailored nutritional programmes that correspond with their unique therapy and medical requirements. A well-designed diet may complement cancer therapy and boost the body's capacity to adapt to treatment.

However, it's vital to note that nutrition alone cannot cure cancer, and it should never substitute normal medical therapies. Instead, it functions as a supporting approach to assist enhance general health and well-being throughout the cancer experience. Always contact with healthcare specialists for suitable recommendations customised to particular circumstances.

2. **Nutritional Needs During Cancer Treatment**

During cancer treatment, keeping good nutrition is vital to support the body's capacity to deal with the difficulties of the illness and its therapies. Here are some basic dietary advice for cancer patients:

1. Sufficient Calories: Cancer and its therapies might raise the body's energy demands. Consuming adequate calories is vital to avoid weight loss and maintain energy levels.

2. Protein Intake: Protein is necessary for tissue repair and the immunological system. Including sources of lean protein such chicken, fish, tofu, beans, and nuts is suggested.

3. Hydration: Staying hydrated is crucial, particularly during treatments that may induce dehydration. Aim to drink lots of water throughout the day.

4. Fruits and Vegetables: These give critical vitamins, minerals, and antioxidants that boost the immune

system and general health. A vibrant variety is preferable.

5. Whole Grains: Choose whole grains like brown rice, whole wheat, quinoa, and oats for their greater fiber content and nutritional benefits.

6. Healthy Fats: Include sources of healthy fats like avocados, nuts, seeds, and olive oil, which are helpful for general health.

7. Manage adverse Effects: Cancer therapies might produce adverse effects including nausea, mouth sores, or trouble swallowing. Opt for softer or liquid meals as required, and work with a dietician to locate acceptable alternatives.

8. Limit Processed meals: Minimize intake of processed and sugary meals, since they give little nutritional value and may significantly effect general health.

9. Consider Supplements: In certain situations, cancer patients may require supplements to satisfy their nutritional demands. Consult with healthcare specialists before using any supplements.

It's crucial to remember that every individual's nutritional demands throughout cancer treatment might differ, based on their exact diagnosis, treatment plan, and general health. Working with an expert registered dietitian or healthcare team is vital to design a tailored nutrition plan that best fits the patient's particular condition.

3. Addressing Common Eating Challenges

Addressing frequent dietary problems during cancer treatment is vital to guarantee appropriate nutrition and improve overall well-being. Here are some solutions to solve these challenges:

1. Nausea and Loss of Appetite: Eat smaller, more frequent meals and try bland or cold foods that may be easier to handle. Avoid strong-smelling or fatty meals. Consider anti-nausea drugs as given by your healthcare professional.

2. Taste Changes: Experiment with various spices and marinades to improve the taste of dishes. Cold or frozen meals could be more pleasant.

3. Mouth Sores: Choose soft, smooth, and lukewarm meals. Avoid acidic, spicy, or crunchy meals that may irritate the mouth. Sucking on ice chips or popsicles may be calming.

4. Difficulty Swallowing: Opt for soft or pureed meals, and try adding sauces or

gravies to moisten them. Avoid dry, gritty, or sticky foods.

5. Fatigue: Plan meals ahead of time, and ask for assistance with meal preparation if required. Include easy-to-eat healthful selections.

6. Dehydration: Drink little quantities of water throughout the day. Infuse water with natural tastes like cucumber or lemon to make it more appetising.

7. Digestive Issues: Eat smaller, frequent meals and avoid big, heavy meals. Consider items that are easy on the stomach, such as simple rice, bananas, or toast.

8. Weight Loss: Opt for high-calorie, nutrient-dense meals. Add healthy fats to meals, such as avocado, almonds, or olive oil.

9. Emotional Eating: Seek counselling from a counselor, therapist, or support group to deal with emotional eating difficulties at this tough time.

10. Dietary Modifications: Work with a trained dietitian to establish a tailored food plan that matches your individual requirements and interests.

Remember, it's vital to discuss honestly with your healthcare provider about any dietary issues you're having. They may give direction, make modifications to your treatment plan if appropriate, and provide extra assistance to help you handle these issues successfully.

CHAPTER TWO

Building a Cancer-Friendly Pantry

1. Stocking Nutrient-Rich Staples

Stocking up on nutrient-rich staples is a good strategy to ensure you have a range of healthy and nutritious meals easily accessible. Here are some nutrient-rich basics to consider keeping in your cupboard and fridge:

1. Whole Grains: Brown rice, quinoa, oats, whole wheat pasta, and whole grain bread give fiber, vitamins, and minerals.

2. Beans and Legumes: Such as black beans, chickpeas, lentils, and kidney beans are good sources of protein, fiber, and different minerals.

3. Nuts and Seeds: Almonds, walnuts, chia seeds, flaxseeds, and pumpkin seeds give healthful fats, protein, and critical elements.

4. Healthy Fats: Avocado, olive oil, and coconut oil are healthful alternatives for cooking and seasoning meals.

5. Canned Fish: Tuna, salmon, and sardines are rich in omega-3 fatty acids and protein.

6. Fruits: Stock up on a variety of fresh, frozen, or canned fruits including berries, oranges, apples, and peaches for vitamins and antioxidants.

7. veggies: Opt for fresh or frozen veggies like spinach, broccoli, carrots, and bell peppers to guarantee a healthy combination of vitamins and minerals.

8. Dairy or Plant-Based Alternatives: Choose low-fat milk, yogurt, or dairy-free choices enriched with calcium and vitamin D.

9. Eggs: A varied source of protein and important minerals.

10. Lean Proteins: Chicken, turkey, tofu, and tempeh are good protein sources.

11. Herbs and Spices: Enhance the taste of your foods with herbs and spices like basil, turmeric, garlic, and ginger, which also provide possible health advantages.

12. Nutritious Beverages: Stock up on water, herbal teas, and natural fruit juices without added sugars.

Remember to store perishable foods properly and check expiry dates often. Having a well-stocked pantry with nutrient-rich basics guarantees you can produce balanced and satisfying meals even on busy days or through hard times. Don't forget to supplement these essentials with fresh food whenever feasible to enhance your nutritional intake.

2. Optimal Food Choices for Cancer Patients

Optimal meal choices for cancer patients concentrate on delivering vital nutrients to enhance general health and well-being throughout treatment. Here are some recommendations:

1. Fruits and Vegetables: Rich in vitamins, minerals, and antioxidants, they help enhance the immune system. Choose a range of colorful alternatives including berries, leafy greens, citrus fruits, and cruciferous veggies.

2. Whole Grains: Brown rice, quinoa, oats, and whole wheat products include fiber, which assists in digestion and gives continuous energy.

3. Lean Proteins: Include sources including chicken, turkey, fish, tofu, and lentils to assist tissue regeneration and immunological function.

4. Healthy Fats: Avocado, nuts, seeds, and olive oil are good sources of healthy fats, which enhance nutrient absorption and offer energy.

5. Dairy or Plant-Based Alternatives: Choose low-fat milk or dairy-free choices enriched with calcium and vitamin D for bone health.

6. Hydration: Drink lots of fluids to keep hydrated, such as water, herbal teas, and natural fruit juices without added sugars.

7. Foods Rich in Omega-3 Fatty Acids: Cold-water fish like salmon, flaxseeds, and walnuts include these healthy fats, which may help decrease inflammation.

8. Small, Frequent Meals: Eating smaller, more frequent meals may help moderate hunger and reduce exhaustion during therapy.

9. Foods High in Vitamin C: Citrus fruits, strawberries, and bell peppers may assist in iron absorption and strengthen the immune system.

10. Soft and Easy-to-Swallow meals: For people with mouth sores or trouble swallowing, try soft, pureed, or liquid meals.

11. Limit Processed Foods and Added Sugars: Minimize processed and sugary foods that give little nutritious benefit.

12. Consult with a Dietitian: Work with a registered dietitian specialised in oncology to design a customised food plan suited to your individual requirements and therapy.

Remember that each person's dietary requirements may differ based on their kind of cancer, treatment regimen, and general health. It's vital to work with healthcare specialists to establish a diet that best meets the individual's particular circumstances.

3. Selecting Healthful Cooking Oils and Ingredients

When picking healthy cooking oils and ingredients, it's crucial to emphasise those that give nutritional advantages and enhance general well-being. Here are some guidelines for selecting nutritious choices:

Healthful Cooking Oils:

1. Extra Virgin Olive Oil: Rich in monounsaturated fats and antioxidants, it's a heart-healthy option for sautéing and salad dressings.

2. Avocado Oil: High in monounsaturated fats, it has a high smoke point, making it excellent for high-heat culinary techniques like frying.

3. Coconut Oil: While it includes saturated fats, utilising virgin coconut oil in moderation may provide a distinct taste to recipes.

4. Canola Oil: Low in saturated fat and rich in monounsaturated fat, it's a flexible alternative for cooking and baking.

5. Grapeseed Oil: A excellent source of polyunsaturated fats, it has a higher smoke point and may be utilised for many cooking techniques.

Healthful Cooking Ingredients: 1. Herbs and Spices: Use a variety of herbs and spices like basil, turmeric, oregano, and cinnamon to add flavor to foods without depending on excessive salt or sugar.

2. Fresh Produce: Incorporate enough of fruits and vegetables in your meals to give critical vitamins, minerals, and antioxidants.

3. Whole Grains: Choose whole grains like brown rice, quinoa, oats, and whole wheat to enhance fiber intake and help digestion.

4. Lean Proteins: Include sources including skinless chicken, fish, tofu, and lentils to offer vital amino acids and assist tissue repair.

5. Nuts and Seeds: Add almonds, walnuts, chia seeds, flaxseeds, and

pumpkin seeds for healthy fats and protein.

6. Low-Fat Dairy or Plant-Based Alternatives: Opt for low-fat milk or dairy-free choices supplemented with calcium and vitamin D.

7. Natural Sweeteners: Use natural sweeteners like honey or maple syrup in moderation instead of processed sugars.

8. Minimize Processed Ingredients: Reduce the usage of processed and packaged foods that are generally heavy in harmful fats, salt, and additives.

9. Balance and Moderation: Focus on a balanced diet with a range of nutrient-rich products while enjoying decadent delights in moderation.

By selecting healthy cooking oils and ingredients, you can produce tasty and nutritious meals that promote your overall health and well-being. Remember to pay attention to portion sizes and practice mindful eating for a well-rounded approach to nutrition.

CHAPTER THREE

Wholesome Breakfasts for Nourishment

1. Nutrient-Packed Smoothies and Shakes

Nutrient-packed smoothies and shakes are a fantastic method to replenish your body with necessary vitamins, minerals, and other helpful elements. Here are some suggestions for preparing nutrient-packed smoothies and shakes:

1. Green Power Smoothie: Ingredients: Spinach or kale, banana, green apple, cucumber, chia seeds, almond milk, and a splash of honey or maple syrup for sweetness.

2. Berry Blast Smoothie: Ingredients: Mixed berries (strawberries, blueberries,

raspberries), Greek yogurt or plant-based yogurt, almond milk, a spoonful of almond butter, and a sprinkle of crushed flaxseeds.

3. Tropical Paradise Shake: Ingredients: Mango, pineapple, coconut milk, Greek yogurt or coconut yogurt, a splash of orange juice, and a scoop of protein powder (optional).

4. Banana Nut Smoothie: Ingredients: Banana, peanut butter or almond butter, low-fat milk or almond milk, a splash of cinnamon, and a handful of walnuts.

5. Chocolate Avocado Shake: Ingredients: Ripe avocado, unsweetened chocolate powder, a dash of vanilla extract, low-fat milk or almond milk, and a natural sweetener like honey or maple syrup.

6. Energizing Blueberry Spinach Shake: Ingredients: Fresh or frozen blueberries,

spinach, Greek yogurt or plant-based yogurt, a spoonful of hemp seeds, and a splash of coconut water.

7. Immune-Boosting Citrus Smoothie: Ingredients: Orange, lemon, plain yogurt or plant-based yogurt, a spoonful of honey, and a slice of fresh ginger.

8. Protein-Packed Green Smoothie: Ingredients: Baby spinach, banana, protein powder (whey or plant-based), low-fat milk or almond milk, and a spoonful of almond butter.

9. Creamy Cherry Almond Shake: Ingredients: Cherries (fresh or frozen), almond milk, plain yogurt or plant-based yogurt, and a teaspoon of almond extract.

10. Superfood Antioxidant Shake: Ingredients: Acai berries (frozen puree or powder), mixed berries, Greek yogurt

or plant-based yogurt, a spoonful of chia seeds, and coconut water.

Feel free to personalise these smoothies and shakes depending on your taste preferences and nutritional requirements. You may add ice cubes, modify the sweetness, or mix additional fruits and veggies to make your preferred nutrient-packed blend. Remember to keep an eye on portion sizes and avoid adding excessive quantities of sweets or high-calorie components to maintain a balanced and wholesome shake or smoothie. Enjoy these nutrient-rich sweets as a pleasant and healthful complement to your diet!

2. Energizing Breakfast Bowls

Energizing breakfast bowls are a terrific way to start your day with a surge of energy and critical nutrients. Here are some ideas for producing invigorating breakfast bowls:

1. Acai Bowl:

Base: Acai berry puree or frozen acai packets combined with a dash of almond milk.

Toppings: Sliced bananas, granola, chia seeds, coconut flakes, and a drizzle of honey.

2. Greek Yogurt Breakfast Bowl: Base: Greek yogurt (plain or flavored) combined with a little honey or maple syrup.

Toppings: Fresh berries (strawberries, blueberries, raspberries), sliced almonds, and a sprinkling of cinnamon.

3. Green Smoothie Bowl: Base: Blend baby spinach or kale with a frozen banana and almond milk until smooth.

Toppings: Chopped kiwi, sliced mango, pumpkin seeds, and a handful of goji berries.

4. Quinoa Breakfast Bowl: Base: Cooked quinoa seasoned with a touch of cinnamon and a splash of almond milk.
Toppings: Sliced peaches, chopped walnuts, dried cranberries, and a drizzle of agave syrup.

5. Chia Pudding Bowl: Base: Chia seeds soaked overnight in almond milk or coconut milk.
Toppings: Sliced strawberries, blueberries, shredded coconut, and a dab of almond butter.

6. Tropical Mango Pineapple Bowl:
Base: Blend frozen mango and pineapple with coconut milk until creamy.
Toppings: Sliced bananas, toasted coconut flakes, and a sprinkling of hemp seeds.

7. Banana Almond Breakfast Bowl:
Base: Blend ripe bananas with almond

butter and a dash of almond milk until smooth.
Toppings: Sliced almonds, sliced dates, and a sprinkle of maple syrup.

8. Overnight Oats Bowl: Base: Mix rolled oats with yogurt and milk (dairy or plant-based) and let it rest overnight in the refrigerator.
Toppings: Sliced apples, raisins, a splash of cinnamon, and a sprinkle of flaxseeds.

Remember, the key to an invigorating breakfast bowl is to contain a balance of complex carbs, protein, healthy fats, and a variety of fruits or vegetables. These nutrient-rich combos will deliver continuous energy throughout the morning and help kick-start your day on a positive note. Feel free to experiment with various ingredients and toppings to build your own invigorating breakfast bowl!

3. Whole-Grain Breakfast Ideas

Whole-grain breakfast recipes are a terrific way to start your day with a healthy and substantial meal. Here are some wonderful choices to consider:

1. Whole-Grain bread: - Top whole-grain bread with mashed avocado and a sprinkling of salt and pepper.
- Spread almond or peanut butter over whole-grain bread and add sliced bananas or berries on top.

2. Overnight Whole-Grain Oats: - Prepare overnight oats using rolled oats, chia seeds, Greek yogurt, and milk (dairy or plant-based). Add your favorite fruits and nuts for added taste and texture.

3. Whole-Grain Pancakes or Waffles: - Make pancakes or waffles using whole-grain flour (such as whole wheat

or oat flour). Top them with fresh fruit and a dab of honey or maple syrup.

4. Quinoa Breakfast Bowl: - Cook quinoa in milk (dairy or plant-based) and add a touch of honey or maple syrup. Top with sliced almonds, dried cranberries, and a dollop of Greek yogurt.

5. Whole-Grain Breakfast Burrito: - Fill a whole-grain tortilla with scrambled eggs, black beans, sliced tomatoes, avocado, and a sprinkling of cheese.

6. Brown Rice Pudding: - Prepare brown rice with milk (dairy or plant-based) and boil until creamy. Add a sprinkle of cinnamon, a handful of raisins, and chopped almonds.

7. Whole-Grain Breakfast Parfait: - Layer Greek yogurt, whole-grain granola, and mixed berries or sliced

fruits in a glass or bowl for a pleasant and healthful breakfast.

8. Whole-Grain Breakfast Muffins: - Bake whole-grain muffins with extra fruits, nuts, or seeds for a portable and filling breakfast choice.

9. Whole-Grain Breakfast Burrito Bowl: - Create a burrito bowl with cooked quinoa, scrambled eggs, sautéed veggies, black beans, and salsa.

10. Whole-Grain Breakfast Cereal: - Opt for whole-grain morning cereals like oatmeal, muesli, or whole-grain bran flakes. Pair them with milk (dairy or plant-based) and fresh fruits.

Whole grains contain fiber, vitamins, minerals, and lasting energy, making them a fantastic option to kick-start your morning. Feel free to mix and match these ideas or get creative with your favorite whole-grain products to create a range of healthful and tasty breakfast alternatives.

CHAPTER FOUR

Nourishing Soups and Healing Broths

1. Immune-Boosting Vegetable Soups

Immune-boosting vegetable soups are a wholesome method to enhance your immune system and keep you healthy. Here are some tasty and nutrient-packed vegetable soup ideas:

1. Hearty Vegetable Soup: - Ingredients: Carrots, celery, onions, tomatoes, zucchini, spinach, and bell peppers.
- Add vegetable broth, garlic, and herbs like thyme, oregano, and bay leaves for flavor.
- You may also incorporate chickpeas or lentils for extra protein and fiber.

2. Immune-Boosting Mushroom Soup:

- Ingredients: A blend of various mushrooms including shiitake, oyster, and button mushrooms.
- Add onions, garlic, vegetable broth, and a dash of tamari or soy sauce for umami flavor.
- Include fresh thyme or rosemary for an extra flavorful touch.

3. Turmeric Carrot Soup: - Ingredients: Carrots, onions, ginger, and turmeric. - Cook in vegetable broth and coconut milk for a creamy texture. - Turmeric is recognised for its anti-inflammatory effects.

4. Spinach and Lentil Soup: - Ingredients: Spinach, red lentils, carrots, celery, and tomatoes.
- Add vegetable broth, garlic, and spices like cumin and paprika.
- Lentils give protein and fiber, while spinach provides important minerals.

5. Cabbage and White Bean Soup: - Ingredients: Cabbage, white beans, onions, and garlic.
- Add vegetable broth, chopped tomatoes, and herbs like thyme and bay leaves.
- Cabbage is rich in vitamins and antioxidants.

6. Roasted Vegetable Soup: - Ingredients: Roasted sweet potatoes, carrots, onions, and garlic. - Blend with veggie broth and a dash of coconut milk for richness.
- Roasting veggies increases their taste.

7. Ginger and Butternut Squash Soup: - Ingredients: Butternut squash, ginger, onions, and vegetable broth.
- Add a sprinkle of nutmeg and coconut milk for a soothing soup.

8. Broccoli and Cauliflower Soup:
- Ingredients: Broccoli, cauliflower, onions, and garlic. - Blend with veggie

broth and a dash of almond milk for a smooth texture.
- Broccoli and cauliflower are filled with vitamins and minerals.

Including a variety of bright veggies in your soups guarantees a broad range of nutrients and antioxidants to help your immune system. Feel free to alter these recipes to fit your taste preferences and nutritional demands. Enjoy these immune-boosting vegetable soups as a tasty and beneficial supplement to your meals.

2. Comforting Bone Broths

Comforting bone broths are not only tasty but also nutrient-rich and relaxing. Here are some traditional and tasty bone broth ideas:

1. Traditional Chicken Bone Broth: - Simmer chicken bones, together with onions, carrots, celery, garlic, and herbs

like thyme and bay leaves, in water for many hours. - The outcome is a pleasant and nutritious soup with a rich chicken taste.

2. Beef Bone Broth: - Roast beef bones before boiling them with onions, carrots, celery, garlic, and herbs like rosemary and parsley. - The slow-cooked beef bone broth is full-bodied and flavorful.

3. Turkey Bone Broth: - After Thanksgiving or a roast turkey meal, use the turkey carcass to prepare a tasty bone broth. - Simmer the turkey bones with onions, carrots, celery, and herbs like sage and thyme for a wonderful broth.

4. Fish Bone Broth: - Use fish bones and heads to produce a delicate and tasty broth.
- Add onions, leeks, carrots, celery, and herbs like dill and parsley to improve the flavour.

5. Vegetable Bone Broth: - Make a vegan-friendly bone broth by utilising a variety of vegetable scraps, such as onion peels, carrot ends, celery leaves, and garlic skins.
- Simmer the vegetable scraps with water and seasonings for a wonderful plant-based broth.

6. Asian-Style Bone Broth: - Create an Asian-inspired bone broth with ginger, garlic, star anise, and cinnamon along with beef or chicken bones. - This fragrant broth is great for soups and noodle meals.

7. Mushroom Bone Broth: - Combine a combination of mushroom stems and vegetable scraps to produce a tasty and umami-rich broth.
- Use it as a foundation for mushroom-based soups and risottos.

Bone broths are not only comfortable to drink on their own but also serve as a terrific basis for many soups, stews, and sauces. They are rich in collagen, amino acids, and minerals, which may be useful for joint health, digestive function, and immunological support. Enjoy these healthy bone broths as a warm and calming complement to your meals!

3. Creamy Pureed Soups for Sensitive Palates

Creamy pureed soups are a good alternative for individuals with sensitive palates, since they are simple to digest and have a smooth texture. Here are some wonderful and soft creamy pureed soup ideas:

1. Creamy Carrot Soup: - Steam or boil carrots until cooked, then combine them with vegetable broth and a dab of

coconut milk for smoothness. Add a sprinkle of nutmeg for added taste.

2. Butternut Squash and Apple Soup: - Roast butternut squash and apples until tender, then combine them with vegetable broth and a splash of maple syrup for sweetness. A sprinkling of cinnamon compliments the taste.

3. Creamy Zucchini Soup: - Cook zucchini with onions and garlic until tender, then purée with vegetable broth and a little cream or almond milk for richness. Fresh basil leaves offer a pleasant touch.

4. Potato Leek Soup: - Sauté leeks and potatoes until soft, then combine with vegetable broth and a dash of milk or dairy-free substitute. Season with thyme and a dash of white pepper.

5. Creamy Cauliflower Soup: - Steam or roast cauliflower until cooked, then

purée with vegetable broth and a little of coconut milk or Greek yogurt. Add a little of turmeric for a golden color and a dab of cumin for warmth.

6. Creamy Tomato Basil Soup: - Cook tomatoes and onions until soft, then combine with vegetable broth and a handful of fresh basil leaves. Stir with a little cream or coconut milk for creaminess.

7. Creamy Spinach Soup: - Cook spinach with onions and garlic until wilted, then purée with vegetable broth and a dash of almond milk. Season with a sprinkle of nutmeg.

8. Sweet Potato and Ginger Soup: - Roast sweet potatoes with ginger until soft, then combine with vegetable broth and a dash of coconut milk or yogurt. A sprinkling of cinnamon provides warmth.

Remember to season your creamy pureed soups with a bit of salt and pepper to taste. These soups are not only mild on delicate palates but also provide a pleasant and nutritional choice for everyone to enjoy. Feel free to alter the recipes to fit your taste preferences and nutritional demands.

CHAPTER FIVE

Flavorful Main Courses for Strength and Vitality

1. Protein-Rich Poultry and Seafood Dishes

Protein-rich poultry and fish recipes provide tasty and healthful alternatives for fulfilling dinners. Here are some suggestions for producing tasty dishes:

Protein-Rich Poultry Dishes:

1. Grilled Chicken Breast: - Marinate chicken breasts in a combination of olive oil, lemon juice, garlic, and herbs before grilling for a moist and tasty main meal.

2. Baked Chicken Thighs: - Season chicken thighs with your preferred spices and herbs, then bake them in the oven until crispy and tender.

3. Chicken Stir-Fry: - Stir-fry sliced chicken with a variety of colorful veggies in a delicious sauce prepared with soy sauce, ginger, garlic, and a bit of honey or brown sugar.

4. Lemon Herb Roast Chicken: - Rub a whole chicken with a combination of lemon zest, garlic, thyme, and rosemary before roasting it in the oven for a wonderful and cosy dinner.

5. Chicken and Vegetable Curry: - Cook chicken pieces with a mix of vegetables in a thick and fragrant curry sauce prepared with coconut milk, curry powder, and spices.

Protein-Rich Seafood Dishes:

1. Grilled Salmon: - Brush salmon fillets with olive oil and season with salt, pepper, and lemon juice before grilling for a tasty and healthful fish entrée.

2. Shrimp Scampi: - Sauté shrimp in garlic, butter, and white wine for a fast and delectable seafood dish.

3. Baked Cod with Herbs: - Coat cod fillets with a combination of herbs including dill, parsley, and thyme, then bake them in the oven until soft and flaky.

4. skillet-Seared Tuna Steaks: - Season tuna steaks with a combination of sesame seeds, soy sauce, and ginger before searing them in a hot skillet for a delightful Asian-inspired meal.

5. Seafood Paella: - Prepare a tasty paella with a mix of shrimp, mussels, clams, and saffron-infused rice for a full and spectacular seafood dinner.

Remember to combine these protein-rich recipes with a range of colorful vegetables, nutritious grains, or salads to produce well-rounded and balanced meals. Whether you favour chicken or fish, these meals provide a varied selection of tastes and cooking ways to enjoy.

2. Plant-Based Protein Alternatives

Plant-based protein alternatives provide a broad choice of tasty and healthy options for people wishing to decrease or remove animal products from their diet. Here are some common plant-based protein sources:

1. Legumes: Beans, lentils, and chickpeas are good providers of protein, fiber, and important minerals.

2. Tofu and Tempeh: Made from soybeans, these adaptable alternatives may be utilised in numerous cuisines and absorb flavors effectively.

3. Edamame: Young, green soybeans are a delightful and protein-rich snack or addition to salads and stir-fries.

4. Seitan: Also known as wheat gluten, it is a high-protein meat replacement with a chewy texture, widely used in plant-based meals.

5. Quinoa: A complete protein containing all nine necessary amino acids, quinoa is a versatile grain that may be used in salads, bowls, or as a side dish.

6. Nuts and Seeds: Almonds, walnuts, chia seeds, hemp seeds, and pumpkin seeds contain protein, healthy fats, and numerous nutrients.

7. Chickpea and Lentil Pastas: These pasta alternatives are richer in protein and fiber compared to typical wheat pasta.

8. Plant-Based Meat Alternatives: Brands provide plant-based burgers, sausages, and other meat alternatives produced from substances like soy, pea protein, or wheat.

9. Nutritional Yeast: A rich source of protein and B-vitamins, it gives a cheesy taste to recipes.

10. Spirulina and Chlorella: These blue-green algae are rich in protein and may be added to smoothies or used as supplements.

11. Plant-Based Milk Alternatives: Some versions of almond, soy, pea, or oat milk are fortified with added protein and vitamins.

12. Spinach and Leafy Greens: While not as protein-dense as some other sources, greens like spinach and kale nevertheless add to protein

consumption and provide various health advantages.

Combining diverse plant-based protein sources may generate well-balanced and healthy meals. Incorporating a variety of legumes, whole grains, nuts, seeds, and plant-based meat substitutes into your diet helps you satisfy your protein requirements while enjoying a broad range of tastes and textures.

3. Delectable Whole Grain Meals

Absolutely! Whole grain dishes may be both delightful and healthful. Here are some delectable ideas for whole grain-based dishes:

1. Quinoa Stuffed Bell Peppers: - Mix cooked quinoa with sautéed veggies, herbs, and spices. - Stuff the mixture into half bell peppers and bake until cooked.

2. Brown Rice Veggie Stir-Fry: - Stir-fry a colorful variety of veggies including broccoli, carrots, bell peppers, and snap peas.
- Toss them with cooked brown rice and a delicious sauce prepared with soy sauce, garlic, and ginger.

3. Spicy Chickpea and Farro Salad: - Cook farro according to package directions and combine it with roasted chickpeas, cherry tomatoes, cucumbers, and chopped herbs.
- Dress the salad with a lemon-tahini dressing for a tangy kick.

4. Lentil and Sweet Potato Curry: - Simmer red lentils with diced sweet potatoes in a coconut milk-based curry sauce seasoned with spices like turmeric, cumin, and coriander.

5. Whole Wheat Pasta Primavera: - Cook whole wheat pasta until al dente

and combine it with a variety of sautéed seasonal vegetables. - Add a light sauce prepared with olive oil, garlic, lemon juice, and fresh herbs.

6. Wild Rice and Mushroom Pilaf: - Cook wild rice and sauté mushrooms, onions, and garlic in a separate pan. - Mix them together and add a bit of vegetable broth, thyme, and a sprinkling of toasted almonds.

7. Bulgur and Chickpea Salad: - Combine cooked bulgur with chickpeas, diced cucumbers, tomatoes, parsley, and mint.
- Dress the salad with a lemon-olive oil vinaigrette for a pleasant and fulfilling supper.

8. Whole Grain Breakfast Bowl: - Create a breakfast bowl using cooked oats, quinoa, or amaranth as the base. - Top it with sliced fruits, nuts, seeds, and a drizzle of honey or maple syrup.

By utilising a range of nutritious grains including quinoa, brown rice, farro, and wild rice, you can make enjoyable dishes with various textures and tastes. Don't forget to include lots of colorful veggies, herbs, and spices to increase the flavour and nutritional content of your food. Enjoy these delightful whole grain meals that feed both your body and taste senses!

CHAPTER SIX

Nutrient-Dense Salads and Side Dishes

1. Fresh and Colorful Salad Combinations

Fresh and colorful salad choices not only look lovely but also deliver a broad variety of nutrients and tastes. Here are some excellent ideas for bright salads:

1. Mediterranean Salad: - Mixed greens, cherry tomatoes, cucumbers, Kalamata olives, red onions, and crumbled feta cheese. - Dress with a simple vinaigrette consisting of olive oil, lemon juice, garlic, oregano, and a bit of salt and pepper.

2. Summer Berry Salad: - Baby spinach or arugula, strawberries, blueberries, raspberries, and toasted almonds.

- Toss with a little honey-lime dressing.

3. Thai Mango Salad: - Shredded green cabbage, ripe mango slices, red bell peppers, carrots, and fresh cilantro. - Drizzle with a dressing prepared from lime juice, soy sauce, sesame oil, and a splash of chile paste.

4. Caprese Salad: - Sliced ripe tomatoes, fresh mozzarella, and basil leaves placed in a circular pattern. - Drizzle with balsamic glaze and extra virgin olive oil.

5. Grilled Vegetable Salad: - Grilled zucchini, eggplant, bell peppers, and asparagus on a bed of mixed greens. - Top with crumbled goat cheese and a balsamic vinaigrette.

6. Mexican Fiesta Salad: - Romaine lettuce, black beans, corn, diced avocado, cherry tomatoes, and cilantro.

- Add a squeeze of lime and a dollop of Greek yogurt as a creamy dressing.

7. Rainbow Quinoa Salad: - Cooked quinoa with a combination of coloured bell peppers, shredded carrots, cherry tomatoes, and fresh parsley. - Dress with a lemon-tahini vinaigrette.

8. Watermelon Feta Salad: - Cubed watermelon, crumbled feta cheese, fresh mint leaves, and a sprinkling of black pepper. - Drizzle with a light honey-lime dressing.

9. Asian Sesame Slaw: - Shredded cabbage, shredded carrots, sliced snow peas, green onions, and toasted sesame seeds. - Toss with a sesame-ginger dressing.

10. Autumn Harvest Salad: - Mixed greens, sliced apples, dried cranberries, candied nuts, and crumbled blue

cheese. - Dress with a maple-balsamic vinaigrette.

Feel free to modify these salads using your favorite toppings and dressings. The secret to a fresh and colorful salad is to utilise a range of seasonal vegetables and add a combination of textures and tastes. Enjoy these refreshing and nutrient-packed salad combos!

2. Wholesome Grain and Legume Salads

Wholesome grain and legume salads are not only tasty but also rich with protein, fiber, and other minerals. Here are some healthful alternatives for grain and legume-based salads:

1. Mediterranean Chickpea and Quinoa Salad: - Cooked quinoa and chickpeas combined with diced cucumbers, cherry

tomatoes, Kalamata olives, red onions, and chopped parsley. - Dress with a lemon-herb vinaigrette prepared with olive oil, lemon juice, garlic, oregano, and a touch of salt and pepper.

2. Black Bean and Brown Rice Salad: - Cooked brown rice and black beans mixed with diced bell peppers, red onions, corn kernels, and chopped cilantro. - Add a tangy dressing with lime juice, cumin, chili powder, and a touch of honey.

3. Lentil and Couscous Salad: - Cooked lentils and couscous blended with sliced carrots, celery, red bell peppers, and fresh mint leaves. - Dress with a lemon-tahini vinaigrette.

4. Quinoa and Edamame Salad: - Cooked quinoa and steamed edamame combined with shredded carrots, sliced green onions, and toasted sesame

seeds. - Toss with a sesame-ginger dressing.

5. Farro and White Bean Salad: - Cooked farro and white beans mixed with roasted cherry tomatoes, baby spinach, and chopped basil. - Dress with a balsamic vinaigrette.

6. Tabbouleh with Red Lentils: - Cooked red lentils combined with diced cucumber, tomatoes, fresh parsley, mint, and bulgur wheat. - Dress with lemon juice, olive oil, and a sprinkle of ground cumin.

7. Wild Rice and Chickpea Salad: - Cooked wild rice and chickpeas blended with diced red onions, dried cranberries, toasted walnuts, and chopped arugula. - Drizzle with a maple-dijon vinaigrette.

8. Three Bean and Barley Salad: - Cooked barley blended with a variety of

kidney beans, black beans, and cannellini beans.
- Add chopped red onions, bell peppers, and a sprinkling of fresh cilantro.
- Toss with a zesty lime-cilantro dressing.

These grain and legume salads are not only healthful and nutritious but also adaptable and enjoyable. Feel free to adjust the ingredients and dressings to suit your taste preferences. Enjoy these tasty salads as a full and beneficial complement to your meals!

3. Vegetable Side Dishes with a Twist

Vegetable side dishes with a twist may bring excitement and new tastes to your meals. Here are some unique methods to improve your veggie dishes:

1. Roasted Cauliflower Steaks: - Slice cauliflower into thick steaks and roast

them with a sprinkle of olive oil, garlic, and your favorite seasonings until they become soft and caramelized.

2. Sweet and Spicy Brussels Sprouts: - Toss halved Brussels sprouts with a combination of honey, sriracha sauce, and a touch of salt before roasting them in the oven for a sweet and spicy bite.

3. Turmeric Roasted Carrots: - Toss entire baby carrots with turmeric, cumin, and a touch of honey or maple syrup before roasting until they are soft and fragrant.

4. Zucchini Ribbon Salad: - Use a vegetable peeler to form thin ribbons of zucchini and mix them with lemon juice, olive oil, fresh basil, and shaved Parmesan cheese.

5. Miso-Glazed Eggplant: - Brush eggplant slices with a miso glaze (prepared from miso paste, soy sauce,

and a bit of brown sugar) before grilling or roasting them to perfection.

6. Cumin and Lime Grilled Corn: - Brush fresh corn on the cob with lime juice and sprinkle ground cumin and chili powder before grilling for a smokey and tangy side dish.

7. Sesame Ginger Green Beans: - Blanch green beans until crisp-tender then combine them with a dressing prepared from sesame oil, ginger, soy sauce, and a sprinkling of sesame seeds.

8. Honey Buttered Asparagus: - Sauté asparagus spears in a combination of honey and melted butter until they are soft and covered with a delicious coating.

9. Cauliflower and Broccoli Popcorn: - Cut cauliflower and broccoli into tiny florets, mix them with olive oil, nutritional

yeast, garlic powder, and salt, then roast until they become crispy and snackable.

10. Chipotle Mashed Sweet Potatoes: - Mash cooked sweet potatoes with chipotle pepper, adobo sauce, and a dash of coconut milk for a spicy and creamy take on classic mashed potatoes.

These innovative vegetable side dishes can bring variety and excitement to your dinners. Feel free to experiment with various flavours, herbs, and sauces to create your own unique spins on basic vegetable dishes. Enjoy the tastes and textures these side dishes offer to your meal!

CHAPTER SEVEN

Managing Eating Challenges During Cancer Treatment

1. Coping with Taste Changes and Loss of Appetite

Coping with taste changes and lack of appetite may be tough, particularly during specific medical treatments or health problems. Here are some ways that may help:

1. Experiment with Different Flavors: Try different seasonings, herbs, and spices to improve the flavour of your dishes. Be open to experiencing new cuisines and taste combinations.

2. Use Aromatics: Strong aromatics like garlic, ginger, and onions may give depth to recipes and boost your appetite.

3. Opt for Cold or Room Temperature meals: Sometimes, cooler or room temperature meals may be more tempting than hot ones.

4. Smaller, Frequent Meals: Instead of three big meals, consider eating smaller, more frequent meals throughout the day to moderate hunger swings.

5. Nutrient-Dense meals: Focus on nutrient-dense meals that contain a lot of nutrients in smaller servings, such as smoothies, soups, and salads.

6. Hydration: Stay hydrated by consuming water throughout the day. You may also try flavored water or herbal teas if plain water seems unattractive.

7. Texture Matters: Experiment with various textures of food to see what is

most appealing for you. Some folks may like crunchy or smooth textures.

8. Seek help: Talk to a healthcare professional or a certified dietitian for tailored guidance and help in managing taste changes and appetite loss.

9. Incorporate Protein: Include protein-rich meals in your diet to assist maintain energy levels and encourage recovery. Plant-based proteins like lentils, tofu, and beans may be easy on the stomach.

10. Mindful Eating: Practice mindful eating by paying attention to the flavour, texture, and fragrance of your meal. This may help you reconnect with your appetite and love of eating.

11. Add Calories to Meals: If your appetite is poor, try adding healthy fats (such avocado, almonds, or olive oil) to

meals to enhance calorie intake without dramatically increasing volume.

12. Avoid Strong odours: Strong odours may sometimes cause taste alterations or diminish appetite. Try to avoid preparing or being around meals with strong scents that may be off-putting.

Remember, it's crucial to be patient and nice to yourself throughout this time. Every person's experience with taste alterations and lack of appetite is unique, so research what works best for you and modify your eating habits appropriately. If these difficulties continue or become serious, it's vital to contact with a healthcare expert to address any underlying concerns.

2. **Tips for Dealing with Nausea and Digestive Discomfort**

Dealing with nausea and intestinal pain may be hard, but there are some ways that may help ease these symptoms. Here are some suggestions to consider:

1. Eat Small, regular Meals: Instead of huge meals, consider eating smaller, more regular meals throughout the day to lessen the load on your digestive system.

2. remain Hydrated: Sip on clear fluids like water, herbal teas, or electrolyte drinks to remain hydrated. Avoid drinking significant quantities of fluids during meals, since it may aggravate feelings of fullness.

3. Avoid cause items: Identify any items that cause your nausea or discomfort, and attempt to avoid them until your symptoms improve.

4. Try Bland meals: Stick to bland, easy-to-digest meals such plain rice,

bread, bananas, applesauce, and boiled potatoes.

5. Ginger: Ginger has inherent anti-nausea effects. Consider ginger tea, ginger sweets, or adding fresh ginger to your meals.

6. Peppermint: Peppermint tea or peppermint oil capsules may help reduce intestinal pain and alleviate nausea.

7. Avoid Strong Smells: Strong scents might provoke or intensify nausea. Stay away from strong-smelling meals and cooking places.

8. Eat Slowly: Take your time when eating and chew your meal properly to help digestion.

9. Keep a Food Diary: Keeping note of what you eat and any symptoms you

feel will help detect trends and possible trigger foods.

10. Stay Upright After Eating: Avoid reclining down shortly after eating. Instead, remain upright for at least 1-2 hours to help avoid acid reflux and indigestion.

11. Relaxation Techniques: Stress and worry may increase intestinal pain. Try relaxing methods like deep breathing, meditation, or moderate yoga.

12. Over-the-Counter Remedies: Over-the-counter antacids or drugs meant to reduce nausea may give brief relief. However, contact with a healthcare expert before taking any drugs.

13. Consult a Healthcare expert: If your symptoms continue or become serious, it's crucial to seek counsel from a

healthcare expert for a thorough examination and specific suggestions.

Remember that everyone's digestive system is different, so it may take some trial and error to discover the best tactics for controlling nausea and digestive pain. Be gentle with yourself and focus self-care at this period.

3. Strategies for Maintaining Hydration

Maintaining hydration is vital for general health and well-being. Here are some proven techniques to help you keep hydrated:

1. Drink Water Regularly: Aim to drink water throughout the day, even if you don't feel thirsty. Carry a reusable water bottle with you to make it easier to remain hydrated.

2. Put Reminders: If you frequently forget to drink water, put alarms or reminders on your phone to push you to take sips regularly.

3. Flavor Water: Add a dash of natural flavor to your water by infusing it with fruits, cucumbers, or mint leaves. This may make drinking water more pleasurable.

4. Eat Hydrating Foods: Include water-rich foods in your diet, such as watermelon, cucumbers, oranges, and celery, which may add to your daily fluid consumption.

5. Drink Before Meals: Have a glass of water before each meal. Not only does this promote hydration, but it may also help reduce hunger.

6. Monitor Urine Color: Pay attention to the color of your urine. Pale yellow or straw-colored urine normally indicates

sufficient hydration, but dark yellow or amber urine may imply dehydration.

7. Avoid Excessive Caffeine and Alcohol: Both caffeine and alcohol may lead to dehydration. If you consume these drinks, drink more water to counteract their diuretic effects.

8. Hydrate During Exercise: Drink water before, during, and after exercise to replenish fluids lost via perspiration.

9. Consider Electrolyte Drinks: In times of extreme physical activity or significant perspiration, consider electrolyte drinks or coconut water to assist replace electrolytes.

10. Monitor Fluid Loss: If you encounter vomiting, diarrhea, or fever, you may lose extra fluids. In such instances, concentrate on consuming clear drinks to preserve hydrated.

11. Create a Hydration regimen: Develop a hydration regimen that corresponds with your everyday routine. For example, you may take a glass of water upon awakening, before meals, and before night.

12. Listen to Your Body: Pay attention to your body's thirst cues. If you feel thirsty, drink water to satisfy your thirst swiftly.

Remember, individual hydration requirements might vary depending on variables such as age, exercise level, and environment. Adjust your fluid intake appropriately to satisfy your body's individual needs. Staying appropriately hydrated helps general health, cognitive function, digestion, and exercise performance.

CHAPTER EIGHT

Indulgent and Nourishing Desserts

1. Healthful Sweet Treats for Sensitive Tastebuds

Healthful sweet snacks for sensitive tastebuds may fulfil your sweet desires while being gentle on your mouth. Here are some wonderful choices to consider:

1. Fruit Sorbet: - Enjoy a delicious and naturally sweet fruit sorbet created from blended frozen fruits like strawberries, mangoes, or peaches.

2. Chia Seed Pudding: - Create a creamy chia seed pudding using chia seeds, your choice of milk (dairy or plant-based), and a natural sweetener

like maple syrup or honey. Top with fresh fruits or nuts.

3. Banana Nice Cream: - Blend frozen bananas till they transform into a creamy and guilt-free ice cream replacement. Add a teaspoon of nut butter or chocolate powder for added taste.

4. Baked Apples: - Core and fill apples with a combination of oats, cinnamon, and a touch of honey or maple syrup. Bake till soft for a warm and naturally sweet delight.

5. Greek Yogurt Parfait: - Layer Greek yogurt with fresh fruits, granola, and a drizzle of honey or agave nectar for a protein-rich and delectable dessert.

6. Dark Chocolate-Covered Berries: - Dip fresh berries like strawberries, blueberries, or raspberries in melted dark chocolate for a delightful sweet treat with antioxidants.

7. No-Bake Energy Bites: - Make no-bake energy snacks using oats, nut butter, honey, and add-ins like chia seeds, shredded coconut, or dried fruits. Roll them into bite-sized balls for a fast and invigorating snack.

8. Baked Pears with Cinnamon: - Slice pears and sprinkle with cinnamon before baking till soft. Serve with a dollop of Greek yogurt for additional creaminess.

9. Date Bliss Balls: - Blend dates, nuts, and a touch of salt until a sticky dough forms. Roll the mixture into bite-sized balls and coat them with shredded coconut or cocoa powder.

10. Rice Cake with Nut Butter and Berries: - Spread nut butter (such as almond or peanut butter) over a rice cake and top it with fresh berries for a simple and tasty dessert.

Remember to alter the sweetness to your taste preferences by adding natural sweeteners like honey, maple syrup, or fruit-based choices. These nutritious sweet delights provide a range of tastes and textures that may appeal to sensitive palettes while supporting a balanced and nourishing diet. Enjoy them guilt-free!

2. Fruit-Forward Desserts with a Touch of Decadence

Fruit-forward sweets with a hint of indulgence provide a lovely blend of sweet and refreshing tastes. Here are some excellent alternatives to quench your sweet tooth:

1. Grilled Peaches with Honey Mascarpone: - Grill ripe peach halves until they have gorgeous grill marks.

- Serve with a dollop of honey-sweetened mascarpone cheese and a sprinkling of toasted almonds.

2. Chocolate-Covered Strawberries with Sea Salt: - Dip fresh strawberries in melted dark chocolate and sprinkle with a sprinkling of sea salt for a sumptuous and balanced treat.

3. Raspberry Lemon Bars: - Prepare conventional lemon bars and top them with fresh raspberries for a tart and vivid variation.

4. Mixed Berry Pavlova: - Create a pavlova with a crispy meringue foundation, topped with whipped cream, and a selection of fresh berries.

5. Mango Coconut Panna Cotta: - Prepare a creamy coconut panna cotta and top it with chopped ripe mangoes for a tropical and delectable dessert.

6. Blueberry Cheesecake Parfait: - Layer crumbled graham crackers, creamy cheesecake filling, and fresh blueberries in a glass for a visually stunning and satisfying dessert.

7. Caramelized Banana Split: - Caramelize ripe banana slices in butter and brown sugar, and then serve with vanilla ice cream, chopped almonds, and a drizzle of chocolate sauce.

8. Baked Apples with Cinnamon Crumble: - Core apples and fill them with a combination of oats, cinnamon, and a touch of honey or maple syrup. Bake till soft and serve with a spoonful of vanilla ice cream.

9. Strawberry Shortcake with Whipped Cream: - Build a traditional strawberry shortcake with layers of fresh strawberries, whipped cream, and soft, buttery shortcakes.

10. Poached Pears in Red Wine: - Poach pears in red wine with cinnamon and cloves until they become soft and filled with rich tastes. Serve with a spoonful of vanilla ice cream or mascarpone cheese.

These fruit-forward sweets provide the right mix between sweetness and the natural tastes of fresh fruits. They are great for indulging in a little luxury while enjoying the benefits of seasonal fruits. Feel free to personalise these desserts using your favorite fruits and toppings to make your fantasy fruit-forward treat!

3. Alternative Ingredients for Traditional Favorites

Alternative components may be utilised to reproduce classic favorite foods, making them appropriate for diverse dietary choices or constraints. Here are some frequent substitutions:

1. Dairy Alternatives: - Use plant-based milk (such as almond, soy, or oat milk) instead of cow's milk in dishes like smoothies, pancakes, and baked goods.
- Replace butter with vegan butter or coconut oil in cooking and baking.

2. Egg Replacements: - Substitute eggs with mashed bananas or applesauce in baking recipes to increase moisture and binding characteristics.
- Use flaxseed or chia seed gel (mix 1 tablespoon of ground flaxseed or chia seeds with 3 tablespoons of water) as an egg replacement in recipes.

3. Gluten-Free Flours: - Use gluten-free flours like almond flour, coconut flour, or a gluten-free baking mix in lieu of wheat flour in recipes.

4. Vegan Protein Sources: - Replace meat with plant-based proteins like tofu, tempeh, seitan, or legumes (such as

chickpeas, lentils, and black beans) in meals like stir-fries, curries, and salads.

5. Cauliflower Rice: - Use grated or processed cauliflower as a lower-carb substitute to rice in meals like fried rice, stir-fries, and grain bowls.

6. Zucchini Noodles (Zoodles): - Spiralize zucchini into noodles and use them in lieu of regular pasta in recipes like spaghetti, pad Thai, or pesto pasta.

7. Nutritional Yeast: - Substitute nutritional yeast for cheese to lend a cheesy taste to foods, such sprinkling it over pasta or popcorn.

8. Coconut Aminos: - Use coconut aminos as a soy sauce replacement in marinades, sauces, and stir-fries for a gluten-free and lower-sodium choice.

9. Date Syrup or Maple Syrup: - Replace refined sugars with natural sweeteners

like date syrup or pure maple syrup in sweets and sweet dishes.

10. Avocado: - Use mashed avocado as a creamy alternative for mayonnaise or as a healthy fat replacement in various recipes.

These alternate components may make classic favorite recipes more inclusive and flexible for varied dietary demands. When making substitutes, bear in mind that the flavour and texture may differ somewhat from the original, so feel free to tweak and experiment until you discover the exact mix that meets your tastes.

CHAPTER NINE

Food and Wine Pairings for Cancer Patients

1. Sensory Experiences to Elevate Mealtime

Elevating meals via sensory experiences may make eating more joyful and memorable. Here are some methods to increase the sensory components of your meals:

1. Visual Appeal: - Present your food with attention to plating and aesthetics. Use bright foods and arrange them attractively on the platter.

2. Aromatherapy: - Incorporate fragrant herbs and spices in your cooking to fill the air with wonderful fragrances that promote hunger.

3. Soft Background Music: - Play soft and pleasant background music at dinner to create a relaxed mood.

4. Natural Light: - Whenever feasible, dine in natural light, as it may improve the eating experience and create a more appealing ambience.

5. Texture Variety: - Include items with varied textures in your meal to give a nice contrast. Combine crunchy, creamy, and chewy characteristics.

6. Engage in Mindful Eating: - Take the time to appreciate each mouthful, paying attention to the tastes and sensations. Be present and totally involved in the meal experience.

7. Use Beautiful tableware: - Use appealing and high-quality tableware, such as colorful plates, exquisite

glasses, and trendy silverware, to enrich the whole experience.

8. Involve All Senses: - Think about the noises of cooking, the perfume of the meal, the appearance of the presentation, the taste, and the textures — engage all your senses.

9. Explore different tastes: - Experiment with different foods and cuisines to discover unique tastes and extend your culinary horizons.

10. Family or Friends Gathering: - Mealtime may be more pleasurable when shared with loved ones. Organize a family or friends gathering to make it a social event.

11. Candlelight Dinners: - Light some candles throughout supper to create a pleasant and intimate mood.

12. Fresh Flowers: - Place fresh flowers or a small potted plant on the dining table to bring a touch of nature to the atmosphere.

13. Memory-Enhancing Foods: - Include foods that recall joyful memories or are connected with positive experiences.

Remember, lunch is not only about sustenance but also about the experience and relationship. By combining these sensory aspects, you may enhance your meals and make it a more fun and fulfilling affair.

2. Wine Selections that Complement Cancer-Friendly Dishes

When picking wine to compliment cancer-friendly recipes, it's necessary to consider the patient's specific health and treatment state. Some cancer treatments and drugs may mix with alcohol, so it's vital to contact with the patient's healthcare team before providing wine. Additionally, some cancer patients may have dietary limitations or allergies, so it's crucial to adjust the food and beverage selections to their unique requirements.

If wine is considered suitable and the patient loves it, here are some basic tips for picking wine that may compliment cancer-friendly dishes:

1. Light to Medium-Bodied Whites: - Opt for light to medium-bodied white wines like Sauvignon Blanc, Pinot Grigio, or Albariño to pair with shellfish, salads, and vegetable dishes.

2. Rosé Wines: - Rosé wines may be adaptable and pair nicely with a variety of foods, from grilled chicken to light pasta dishes.

3. Light-Style Red Wines: - Look for light red wines like Pinot Noir or Gamay to match poultry, mushroom dishes, and lighter meats.

4. Low Alcohol concentration: - Choose wines with lower alcohol concentration, since they may be kinder on the taste and body.

5. Sparkling Wines: - Sparkling wines like Champagne or Prosecco may be great partners to appetizers, shellfish, and fruit-based desserts.

6. Organic or Biodynamic Wines: - If feasible, try buying organic or biodynamic wines that are produced with less interference and fewer ingredients.

It's vital to note that each person's taste preferences varies, and wine choices may be quite distinctive. Always emphasise the patient's well-being and happiness while making any eating selections.

If the patient is not able to drink alcohol or prefers non-alcoholic choices, there are various alcohol-free alternatives available, such as non-alcoholic wines, sparkling water with fruit infusions, or alcohol-free cocktails. These solutions may nevertheless deliver a distinctive and delightful eating experience. Again, speak with the patient's healthcare team for individualised counsel based on their unique medical condition and treatment plan.

3.   Mindful Consumption for Enhanced Enjoyment

Mindful consumption is about being present and completely involved in the experience of eating, which may lead to improved pleasure and a deeper connection with your food. Here are some strategies for practicing mindful consumption:

1. Slow Down: Take your time to eat, relish each mouthful, and chew your meal fully. This helps you to properly taste and enjoy the flavors.

2. Engage Your Senses: Pay attention to the fragrance, texture, and look of the meal. Engage all your senses to thoroughly appreciate the dish.

3. Limit Distractions: Avoid eating while watching TV, looking through your phone, or working. Create a peaceful and concentrated setting for your meal.

4. Appreciate the Source: If feasible, learn about the origin of the components and the cooking procedure. Understanding the work that goes into your food might boost your enjoyment.

5. Express thanks: Take a minute to express thanks for the food on your plate and all the individuals involved in delivering it to you.

6. Mindful food Control: Be mindful of food sizes and heed to your body's hunger signals to prevent overeating.

7. Notice Your Hunger Levels: Before eating, check in with yourself to measure your hunger level. Are you actually hungry, or is there another reason you desire to eat?

8. Pause Between Bites: Set your utensils down between bites and take a minute to breathe. This may avoid mindless eating and help you to gauge your pleasure level.

9. Practice Non-Judgment: Be gentle to yourself and avoid judgment about what or how much you're eating. Embrace a

non-critical attitude towards your eating choices.

10. Be Open to New Experiences: Try new meals or variants of recipes to extend your culinary horizons and experience diverse sensations.

11. Listen to Your Body: Pay attention to how your body reacts to various meals. Notice how particular meals make you feel physically and emotionally.

12. Cultivate Mindful Cooking: Extend attention to the cooking process by appreciating the preparation and handling of materials with care.

Practicing mindful consumption may lead to a greater appreciation of food and a more fulfilling dining experience. By being present and attentive at meals, you may develop a healthy connection with food and feed both your body and mind.

CHAPTER TEN

Nurturing the Mind-Body Connection

1. Emphasizing Mindfulness in Food Preparation and Consumption

Emphasizing mindfulness in food preparation and consumption may improve the way you experience meals and lead to a more pleasant and happy relationship with food. Here are some methods to include mindfulness into your dietary journey:

1. Mindful Meal Planning: Take time to prepare your meals consciously, considering a balance of nutrients and tastes. Include a mix of colorful fruits, veggies, nutritious grains, and lean meats.

2. Connect with Ingredients: When shopping for groceries, take a time to connect with the ingredients. Notice their colors, textures, and fragrances, and enjoy the sustenance they will bring.

3. Engage the Senses: While cooking, engage all your senses. Listen to the sizzling of ingredients, smell the scents, and feel the textures. This increases the cooking experience and anticipation of the dinner.

4. Practice appreciation: As you prepare your meals, develop appreciation for the food, the people engaged in its creation, and the chance to feed yourself and others.

5. Cooking as Meditation: View cooking as a type of meditation. Focus on the work at hand, keeping present with each action and component.

6. Mindful Food Chopping: When chopping vegetables or herbs, stay alert to the rhythmic action and the sound of the knife striking the cutting board.

7. Slow Down While Eating: Eat slowly and digest your meal completely. Take time to taste and savour each mouthful, noticing the tastes and textures.

8. stop Before Digging In: Before taking your first bite, take a minute to stop and show appreciation for the food in front of you.

9. Eliminate Distractions: Avoid distractions like screens or other activities at meals. Create a setting where you can totally concentrate on your meal.

10. Listen to Your Body: Pay attention to hunger and fullness signs. Eat when you are hungry, and quit when you are content.

11. Practice Mindful Eating: Mindful eating entails eating with purpose and attention. Be interested about your eating patterns and feelings surrounding food.

12. Reflect on Your event: After the dinner, take a minute to reflect on the event. Notice how you feel physically and emotionally after eating attentively.

By prioritising mindfulness in food preparation and consumption, you may establish a deeper connection with your food and develop a higher understanding of your body's requirements. This strategy develops a better and more enjoyable connection with food, leading to greater well-being and enjoyment with your meals.

2. Creating a Calming Environment for Mealtime

Creating a peaceful setting for lunch may improve your dining experience and encourage relaxation as you eat. Here are some ways to assist you build create a peaceful atmosphere:

1. Choose a Quiet Setting: Select a pleasant and quiet spot for your dinner. Avoid situations with distractions like loud sounds or heavy traffic.

2. Soft Lighting: Opt for soft, warm lighting rather than strong, harsh lights. Candles or subdued lighting may create a peaceful environment.

3. Mindful Table Setting: Set the table deliberately with clean and elegant dishes. Use relaxing colors and textures to produce a feeling of tranquillity.

4. comfy Seating: Use comfy seats or cushions to guarantee that you can relax and enjoy your meal without pain.

5. Declutter the place: Clear any superfluous materials or clutter from the dining area to create a clean and peaceful place.

6. Background Music: Play gentle and relaxing background music if you find it comforting. Choose instrumental or natural sounds to eliminate distractions.

7. Mindful Breathing: Take a few deep breaths before beginning your meal to center yourself and reduce any remaining stress or tension.

8. Mindful thankfulness: Begin the meal with a moment of thankfulness or a brief mindful meditation to bring your focus to the present moment.

9. Practice Mindful Eating: Slow down your eating rate, chew your meal properly, and appreciate each mouthful consciously. Focus on the tastes and textures of the meal.

10. No displays Allowed: Avoid using phones, iPads, or other displays at meals. This permits you to be totally present with your food and your dining partners.

11. Nature-Inspired Decor: Incorporate natural items like fresh flowers or potted plants to provide a feeling of nature into your mealtime atmosphere.

12. Invite Loved Ones: Sharing a meal with loved ones may provide a feeling of warmth and connection, adding to a tranquil ambiance.

Remember, the tranquil setting you create for eating should represent your unique tastes and requirements. By setting up a calm atmosphere, you may completely immerse yourself in the eating experience and discover greater pleasure and relaxation throughout your meals.

3. Incorporating Gentle Exercise and Movement

Incorporating light exercise and movement into your daily routine may be excellent for general health and well-being. Here are some options for combining mild activities:

1. Walking: Take frequent walks in your neighborhood or a nearby park. Walking is a low-impact activity that benefits cardiovascular health and may be done at your own speed.

2. Yoga: Practice mild yoga or chair yoga to increase flexibility, balance, and relaxation. Yoga may be customised to

suit various fitness levels and physical attributes.

3. Tai Chi: Consider practising tai chi, a graceful and flowing martial art that increases balance, coordination, and stress reduction.

4. Stretching: Incorporate regular stretching activities to enhance flexibility and minimise muscular strain.

5. Dancing: Enjoy dancing to your favorite music at home. It's a great way to exercise your body and raise your attitude.

6. Swimming: If you have access to a pool, swimming is a low-impact activity that is gentle on the joints and delivers a full-body workout.

7. horticultural: Engage in horticultural tasks including planting, weeding, and watering. Gardening may be relaxing

and a fantastic way to connect with nature.

8. riding: Consider modest riding on a stationary bike or tricycle to enhance cardiovascular health and leg strength.

9. Mindful Breathing Exercises: Incorporate mindful breathing exercises or meditation into your everyday routine to decrease stress and improve relaxation.

10. Balance Exercises: Perform balance exercises like standing on one leg or using a balance board to strengthen stability and avoid falls.

11. domestic duties: Engage in light domestic duties like cleaning, vacuuming, or washing dishes. These exercises give a chance to move and burn calories.

12. Active activities: Pursue activities that entail mild movement, such as painting, ceramics, or gentle dancing.

Remember to start cautiously and listen to your body. It's crucial to pick activities that suit your fitness level and any physical constraints you may have. If you have any health concerns or medical issues, contact with your healthcare professional before starting any workout regimen. Incorporating light exercise and movement into your daily routine may contribute to increased physical and emotional well-being, making it a fun and gratifying aspect of your lifestyle.

THANKS